The Ultimate Six Pack Abs Guide

by Neo Monefa

Table of Contents

1. Introduction

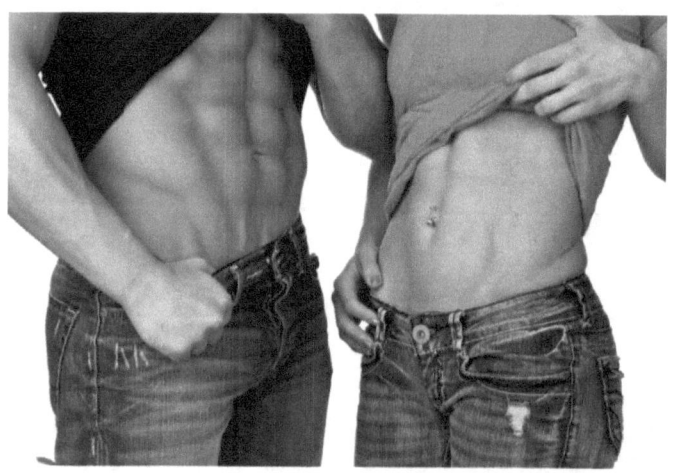

Ever wondered how those male models on the cover of men's magazines get their ripped abs? Or what on earth did they do to develop those six-packs? We always hear men vowing to commit to the gym until they form rock hard abs of their own. But do they really know what they are doing?

Before we plunge head on to the world of better fitness, let us first discuss what those abs really are. They are the stomach muscles running along both sides of our abdomen that keep our body upright. In other words, they are our body's core, so it is indeed logical to fully develop and strengthen them as it is used for all the other exercises. Much more than that, sporting a six-pack is practically a declaration of a person's dedication to being healthy.

Developing Abs and Losing Fat

Building a six-pack requires losing fat. Fat that are stored in the abdomen area are usually very hard to burn away, so a person who wants to develop his abs muscles has to make a drastic change to an unhealthy diet. That means one's eating habits should be leaning towards a lot of protein and smaller portions of fat and carbohydrates. This will be explained further in chapter four.

Abdominal muscles can be fully developed through 3 major factors, namely proper nutrition plan, exercise and supplements. And this cannot be emphasized often and hard enough, but diet is the most important factor, probably accounting for 90% of the reason for ripped abs. Of course, genes may also be a factor, but so long as one follows a healthy nutrition plan complemented with the right training program and vitamins and supplements, then a six-pack is definitely achievable.

The Major Abdominal Muscles You Need to Develop

1. Rectus Abdominals

It is a long and flat muscle running down your body. The middle looks like it has a canal, and there are 3 parallel separations as well.

This is the muscle that makes six-pack abs look ripped and rock hard.

This muscle helps in stretching out our spinal cord. It is the muscle utilized when you bend from one side to another. It also supports the torso's movement.

Any abdominal exercise will work out the rectus abdominals thoroughly.

2. External Obliques

This is a pair of abdominal muscles that form a letter V from the pelvis to the ribs. All abdominal exercises will affect the external obliques, but if you want to focus on it and intensify its effect, do exercises that will circumrotate the abdomen, like twisting crunches and twisting leg raise. Turning to the right will create tension on the left external oblique, and vice versa.

3. Internal Obliques

A pair of deeper lying abdominal muscles located just below the external obliques. It is the opposite of the external obliques in the sense that it looks like an inverted V, straddling from the base of the pelvis to the ribs. The same exercises can be used, though the effect will be the opposite to that of the external oblique. Turning to the right will exercise the right internal oblique, and turning to the left will affect the left internal oblique.

The rectus abdominals, external obliques and internal obliques, along with the transverse abdominals, are the muscles that support and manipulate our body's backbone. Together with the muscles in our lower back region, they form the muscles that connect the upper body to the lower body. Collectively, these muscles are known as our body's core.

Abs training is necessary to build up a strong and powerful core that is important if you want to perform dynamic and athletic movements. A strong core also helps prevent back pain. It will allow you to stand a bit taller literally and figuratively in all aspects of life.

2. Six Pack Secrets

Step 1 – A Lifestyle Check

Before we even begin the serious task of achieving ripped abs, it may be wise to know that attaining a six-pack will entail commitment on your part. You must have both the time and the energy so that you can strictly monitor your diet and food intake and so that you can do the necessary exercises and training. This will probably mean an adjustment in your lifestyle so that you can attain the goal that you have set out for.

It is also important to emphasize that you need to get the right amount of sleep and that you reduce the level of stress in your life. Innocuous as it may seem, these are significant if you are to reach proper fitness that will lead to ripped-up abs.

Step 2 – The Nutritional Requirement of Six-Pack Abs

The most important step in ripping up your abs to show off a six-pack is changing your diet. The key here is controlling insulin, which is the major hormone used in storing body fat. The usual and immediate reaction to this is taking a diet that is low in fat. This is not necessarily true however. Controlling your insulin level means a nutrition program that may be moderate in fat (but low in the saturated kind and absolutely none of the transfat), so long as it is high in protein and low in carbohydrates. This is what we call an abs-friendly diet.

There may be exceptions to this rule, of course. Athletes in their prime can usually consume food high in carbohydrates as they burn these things off quite easily. For most of us however, hunger intensity can be managed a lot better with a low carbohydrate nutrition program.

It is also advisable to eat more frequently but in smaller sizes. Consuming several meals in a day can actually drive your metabolism, which in turn will burn more calories.

Speaking of calories, make sure that you are taking in less than what you are burning. Always check the calorie size of your meal. Calorie intake can also be lessened when you eat food that are rich in fiber, examples of which include fruits and vegetables, whole grains, and other items that are dense with nutrients.

Lastly, try to drink more water. Sometimes, a growling stomach is just an indication of thirst and the need for fluids.

All these will be discussed more extensively in chapter four.

Step 3 – Getting Physical Through Exercise and Training

Now that you have changed your nutrition program, it is time to take the next step in ripping up your abs. This can be done through regular exercise and weight training. Do it correctly by following a program. Don't overdo things by lifting weights or exercising every single day. On the contrary, everyday training may prove to be counterproductive.

Remember to do warm-ups before each exercise to prepare your muscles. Make sure also to consume plenty of liquids in between exercise sets.

A 30- to 60-minute cardio workout three to five times a week must be included. See what cardio exercise you like or will fit you the most. It is very important that you enjoy your workouts so that you will see it to its end. The intensity of your cardio training must also be varied from time to time so that you will get the most out of your workouts.

Weight training should also be incorporated into your exercise program. While the ultimate aim is to achieve a six-pack, conduct your weight training so that it will target all your muscle groups and not just your abs. This should be done twice or thrice a week, but on non-consecutive days.

Try training with exercise balls as well. Abs can be made to work more strenuously in any exercise that tests and challenges your stability. Working out with exercise balls is the perfect answer to this.

As simple as it may sound, exercises involving isometric contractions can also help. Contracting your abs and maintaining it while flexed will help with muscle memory. Develop this habit and soon enough, you will find that you are contracting your abs without consciously doing it. This will show off your six-pack even more.

After your workouts, make sure that you do stretching cool downs to help you relax and achieve more flexibility.

Training exercises are discussed in detail in chapter five.

3. The Fat Burning Process

As mentioned in an earlier chapter, developing a six-pack entails losing those hard to burn fat surrounding the abdominal area. But why do we really need to do this? How is this done?

The Science in the Process of Burning Fat

Fat is a source of energy for our body. The only problem is that they are just the secondary source. The glucose supplied by carbohydrates is the primary source.

So what needs to be done is to burn away those fats. In order to do that, the body has to lose calories first. Burning away even just a single pound of fat would require losing 3,500 calories.

Does that mean we should lessen our calorie intake? Now, don't go crazy and start with one of those extremely low calorie diets. The body needs calories to sustain it, so starving yourself with low calorie meals will just make your body respond negatively. The body will merely slow down its metabolism rate, and a slow metabolism rate will lead to a hoarding of fat. Not quite what you want to achieve.

Neither should you go overboard and eat more than your required calorie level. That is the main reason why people gain weight, when they consume food with more calories than they can actually burn.

So stick to just the right amount. And in reducing your calorie level, do it the correct and proper way.

Losing Fat by Going on a Weight Loss Nutrition Program

As mentioned earlier, losing fat require burning calories first. But burning calories must be done in the right way without starving your body. Carbohydrate intake must be reduced and can be done by avoiding pastries, ice cream, white rice, and the like. Instead of carbohydrates, calories should be sourced from protein instead.

Protein will help your muscles retain mass. In addition, the mere act of digesting protein will burn more calories than when you digest an equal amount of carbohydrates.

Fat must also be consumed more moderately. Bear in mind however that the human body needs healthy fat to function properly. Fats from eggs, as well as omega-3 fatty acids, are good for the body.

4. The Food Requirement

A Healthy Nutrition Plan and Meal Options

Monitoring your food intake is the most important aspect if you want to get ripped abs. While training and exercise, as well as supplements, are highly recommended and necessary, you cannot attain a six-pack if you do not follow a correct diet plan.

The following are some of the nutritious options that you may consider. Take note however that it is essential that you do not exceed your calorie allotment for the day. Calorie requirements may vary depending on gender, muscle mass, amount of activity, etc. If you want to lose weight however, it is advisable that you decrease your daily calorie consumption by at least 500 calories. This may be done either by limiting your intake or by exercising to burn it off, or through a combination of both. Daily calorie intake must not drop below 1,200 for women and 1,800 for men.

As a general rule of thumb, the recommended daily calorie requirement can be computed as follows:

- Male – Body weight in kilograms x 24
- Female – Body weight in kilograms x 24 x 0.9

Also, remember that you should always have a breakfast fit for royalty. It is the most essential meal of the day, so make sure that you consume a combination of protein, complex carbs, and healthy fat to jumpstart your metabolism that will fuel your entire day.

Several Meals a Day Weight Loss Strategy

Consuming three square meals a day is a perfectly good way to eat. But do you know that increasing the frequency of your meals could actually help you lose weight?

Eating several small meals in a day can lead to weight loss, aside from improving your metabolism, increasing energy levels and reducing cholesterol. It will also help in maintaining a lean muscle mass.

Try eating around four to six times each day, spacing your meals around two to three hours from each other. These scheduled intervals will also help your body attain a stable sugar level.

Eating more frequently in small quantities can also help your body control hunger. Your body will always have a feeling of fullness, thus, helping prevent the onset of hunger pangs. Note however that if you follow this weight loss strategy, you have to make sure that you are eating in regular interval patterns without skipping any scheduled meals. Missing a meal will mess up a person's metabolism, and the resulting hunger borne out of a missed scheduled meal will just make you want to eat even more.

All the meals should be well balanced with all the required nutrition elements, meaning it must include lean protein, complex carbs, as well as healthy fat. You can also try dividing your calorie requirement evenly into all your small meals.

Healthy Cheat Meals

Following a healthy diet usually means computing every single gram and calorie of each boring and bland-looking and -tasting food that you have to eat. What choice do you have, when this is a necessary step so that you can have ripped abs?

So that you would not lose your mind, you can actually set aside one meal that will allow you to take a break from your nutrition program. This cheat meal will keep your body guessing and your metabolism on its toes. In this meal, you can go a bit unhealthy even for just one time each week.

Just as a sample, you can probably eat something like this:

- Appetizer. You can even indulge yourself in any of those fried stuff. Or maybe a bowl of soup, or salad with sinful dressing.
- Entrée'. You can actually have anything a restaurant has to offer. Pander yourself to what you have been missing the most, be it a steak, or an order of burger and fries, or pizza, etc.
- Dessert. Top it off with one of your guilty pleasures. Get your hands on that banana split you have been craving for, or blueberry cheesecake, or a slice of apple pie.

Remember that this is just a cheat meal, not a cheat day. Enjoy and indulge, but do not overdo it. You must be able to eat normally on your next scheduled meal without any hitch.

Easy Meal Options

One of the main problems in following a healthy nutrition plan is its availability. People usually do not have the time to prepare their own healthy meals. In order to get six-pack abs however, one must have the drive, the discipline and the commitment to follow through. And yes, this includes having the time to prepare your own meal.

5. Simple & Healthy Food Options

Breakfast

Option # 1

Ingredients:

cup of brown rice
1/3 cup of red beans
egg
tablespoon of low fat cottage cheese
teaspoon of chopped cilantro

How to Prepare:

Cook the brown rice. To make it even easier, there are now brown rice products that can be cooked using a microwave oven.
Mix the beans with the brown rice.
Shred the low fat cottage cheese.
Boil the eggs.
Place the eggs, low fat cheese and cilantro on top of the brown rice and beans combo.

This is good for one serving and will provide you with 379 calories only.
Option # 2

Ingredients:

½ banana
cup of low fat milk
½ cup of mixed berries

¾ cup of oatmeal
tablespoon of pecan or almond nuts
tablespoon of plain yogurt
Healthy Breakfast Meals

Oatmeals and egg whites are the usual breakfast of those wanting to lose weight and getting ripped abs. Keep it interesting by putting some variations into it that are equally healthy and will make the food more palatable. You can include with a half cup of oatmeal a serving of whey protein and a tablespoon of natural peanut butter. You can even top it off with some blueberries to give it more texture. If eggs are your thing, however, always remove the yolk and just concentrate on the egg whites.

Here are some more breakfast menus that you may want to consider:
🔲
1 teaspoon of flax seed
1 teaspoon of vanilla whey protein powder

How to Prepare:

Beat the egg vigorously.
Add the low fat milk, the berries, oatmeal, pecan or almond nuts, flax seed and the vanilla whey protein powder.
Cook in the microwave for 2 minutes.
Place the banana and yogurt on top.

This is good for one serving and will provide you with 590 calories only.

Lunch

Option # 1

Ingredients:

¾ cup of precooked cut chicken
1   romaine lettuce
2   tablespoons of onions
2 tablespoons of feta cheese
1 whole wheat tortilla

How to Prepare:

Place everything on the center of the tortilla.
Roll it up as tight as you can.

Grill it for 3 minutes each side.
You can even add some salsa dip for better taste.

This is good for one serving and will provide you with 397 calories only.

Option # 2

Ingredients:

3 cups of mixed green vegetables
2 small apples
2 slices of smoked turkey
1 tablespoon of balsamic vinegar
1   tablespoon of blue cheese
2   tablespoons of carrots
1 ½ tablespoon of dried cranberries
1 tablespoon of pecan nuts
1 ½ teaspoon of olive oil

How to Prepare:

Chop into small pieces the apples, smoked turkey, carrots and pecan nuts.

Mix it with the green vegetables, blue cheese and dried cranberries. Top it with a dressing made out of balsamic vinegar and olive oil.

This is good for one serving and will provide you with 296 calories only.

Healthy Snacks

The easiest snack to consume is shakes made from whey protein. It is simple, requires almost no effort to make, readily available, and fully satisfying. The problem is if you consume this every snack time, it will become boring and unexciting.

Some variation is in order to break this repetitiveness. By simply adding a tablespoon of natural peanut butter and a bit of water, then placing it in the microwave for about a minute, you can now have a brownie with rich protein content.

Below is a list of snack servings with low calories that you may want to consider.

Easy Snack Options
Snacks with serving of up to 200 calories only

- Cottage cheese stick
- Olives
- Peanut butter (Skippy) stick
- Whole grain biscuit crackers, filled with a can of tuna
- 1 cup of berries (blackberries, strawberries or blueberries), topped with yogurt and a tablespoon of low fat granola
- Cinnamon and peaches, topped with a cup of low sodium cheese
- 5 cups of microwave popcorn, with a tablespoon of cheese
- 6 strawberries, dipped in chocolate syrup

Snacks with serving from 201-400 calories only

- Oatmeal with low fat milk, brown sugar, walnuts and a fresh fruit
- ½ cup of garbanzo beans or chickpeas, mashed and mixed with tahini, lemon juice, olive oil, salt, garlic and roasted vegetables
- 1 whole grain bread, with a piece of banana and some natural peanut butter
- 1 whole grain muffin, filled with a combo of natural peanut butter and jelly
- 1 whole grain muffin, topped with melted cheese and filled with one egg

Healthy Fast Food Meals

Fast food is usually associated with fat foods. It has been largely blamed as one of the major causes of obesity. The popular thinking is that if you want to lose weight, burn fat, and get ripped six-pack abs, you should completely cut off the consumption of fast food meals.

There is no denying, however, that fast food items are attractive to the taste buds, easy on the budget, and accessible and available whenever and wherever. So instead of totally rejecting fast food, you should find a way of making it work for you.

We have to set some boundaries first, however. Sweetened sodas, french fries, and other fried foods are definitely off the list. There are healthy substitutes that are low in both fat and calories that you can consider. Sandwiches made of grilled chicken, baked potatoes, and fruit parfaits are good for your body. Burgers can even be consumed, provided that it is not one of those big, over the top, whooper kinds.

Eat less of the toppings and dressings, as they are packed with calories. You can ask the food server to prepare your meal without mayonnaise and those other special sauces. For salad meals, do away with high calorie ranch dressings and use instead vinaigrette dressing.

Healthy Post Workout Meals

Training and exercise must be followed within the next hour by a healthy meal that will help you recover. It is during this period that the muscles are most receptive and the body is most efficient in storing glucose that you will need for energy and in building protein to help your tired muscles. So the meal must be a good combination of protein and starchy carbohydrates.

The easiest snack to grab after a workout session is a piece of fruit that is gulped down with whey protein shake. You can also try eating half a piece of sweet potato with low fat cheese. They are perfect sources of healthy carbohydrates and protein that are ideal after training.

Option # 1

The Recovery Smoothie

Ingredients:

Banana
Milk
Yogurt

How to Prepare:

Place all the ingredients in a blender.
Make a smoothie.

This recovery drink will provide you with protein and carbohydrates, as well as potassium and magnesium.

Option # 2

The Granola Snack

Ingredients:

Granola bars
Low fat yogurt

How to Prepare:

Top the granola with some low fat yogurt.

Eat in moderation because while this snack will provide a boost to your energy, the calorie content may be high.

This snack will provide you with protein, carbohydrates and healthy fat, as well as iron that is good for your red blood cells.

Option # 3

The Salmon Serving

Ingredients:

Salmon
Vegetables
Brown rice

How to Prepare:

Steam the salmon and the vegetables.

Add to brown rice.

This meal has protein, healthy carbohydrates and omega 3 fat that is good for the heart. It also has fiber and vitamin B complex that help produce energy.

6. Diet and Nutrition Tips During the Weight Loss and Abs Ripping Process

The most important thing when trying to lose weight and gaining that six-pack abs is that one must strictly follow and comply with the nutrition plan that has been laid out. It will entail discipline and a lot of commitment, but bear in mind that there is a reason why your diet has been planned that way.

Skipping a meal will not help and is definitely not advisable. Remember that hunger is the best appetizer, so depriving yourself of a scheduled meal will just worsen the situation as there will be a tendency to compensate excessively the next time you see food.

Besides, skipping a meal will just slow down your metabolism rate, which in turn will signal your body to hoard and hold on to your fat. Whatever weight you lose by skipping a meal will just be temporary in nature as this will be mostly in water.

So the most effective way to lose weight is not by skipping a meal, but by eating more frequently in smaller servings. This will train the body for higher metabolism, thus burning your fat and calories every three hours or so.

Nutrition Plan Based on Somatotype (Body Type)

Our bodies were created in different ways, with genetics playing a role as to its shape and type. There are people who can sport an athletic body without even trying, while there are others who tend naturally to be either thin or stout. A diet or nutrition plan can be designed depending on your somatotype that can help your body achieve optimal condition.

Note that what we are planning to do here is to maximize the natural state of your body by working with what you already have. It does not mean however that following a diet plan outside of your somatotype is harmful and dangerous.

Ectomorphs – The Skinny Ones

Those who are naturally thin are called ectomorphs and will have a hard time attaining a prominent muscle mass. Stuff the food in because ectomorphs need those extra calories. An ectomorph must make sure that he involves himself in a training exercise so that the food will go to building muscles instead of becoming fat. Eating several times a day and indulging with generous amounts of protein shakes, fresh fruit juices, yogurt smoothies, nuts and cheese can also help significantly.

Recommended intake is 55% of carbs, 25% protein and 20% fat.

Mesomorphs – The Athletic Types

Mesomorphs are people blessed with good genes. They have naturally athletic bodies who can eat anything so long as it is within the boundaries of a healthy diet. Mesomorphs seldom have problems with losing weight.

Recommended intake is 50% carbs, 30% protein to help muscle mass, and 20% fat.

Endomorphs – The Stout-Bodied Ones

Those who are naturally round are called endomorphs. While gaining muscles can be quick and easy, an endomorphs' diet should be focused on losing weight. Endomorphs must watch their grain intake, and instead focus on fruits, vegetables and lean protein.

Creating a calorie deficit can shake off weight, meaning intake must be a bit below what the body requires.

Endomorphs have a slow metabolism rate, so recommended intake of carbs is only at 45% maximum, while increasing protein to 35% in order to compensate. The rest can come from healthy fat.

7. How Sweet It Is – Consuming Honey for Weight Loss

We seldom associate sweet food items with losing weight. Even those highly touted refined dietary sugars can actually have an opposite effect. They do not really have any vitamins and minerals to speak of, and even worse, they actually make use of nutrients in our body for it to be processed into our system. These nutrients are precious because it could have been otherwise used for the metabolism of cholesterol and fatty acids that end up being stored in our organs and tissues. We thus end up being stouter than before.

But wait, a simple sugar called honey can actually help in your drive to lose weight and gain ripped up abs. Unlike processed sugar that is devoid of nutrients, honey contains a lot of essential vitamins and minerals that can help your body burn even more fat content. Honey is all-natural and contains 22 amino acids, calcium, fluoride, iron, magnesium, manganese, phosphorous, potassium, selenium, vitamin B and vitamin C. Contrast that to processed sugar that only has mere trace amounts of manganese and riboflavin.

Sure, processed sugar has lesser calories. A tablespoon of honey has around 64 calories, as compared to processed sugar that has 49 calories. However, honey is naturally sweeter by around 1.5 times than processed sugar, meaning you will require a smaller serving to sweeten your drink. The net effect is that you will be consuming lesser calories in the end.

So how exactly does it work? Consuming honey speeds up your body's metabolism, meaning you will be burning more fats. Also, honey has been found to promote healthy insulin levels, which in turn will lead to a stable blood sugar level. A stable blood sugar level will leave you with a feeling of satisfaction, thus decreasing your appetite for more food.

But just like any other items in your nutrition plan, always consult a doctor first, especially to those suffering with or has a history of diabetes. Do not feed honey to kids below a year old, as there is a risk of botulism. Also, as with any food you will consume, take it in moderation.

8. Big Things Come from Small Food

Almonds, pine nuts, cashews, walnuts, peanuts, hazelnuts, pistachios – these are all nuts. Pumpkin seeds, sunflower seeds and sesame seeds – these are seeds that are equally healthy for you.

Nuts and seeds are small food items that are easy to munch on and eat. They only have a small amount of saturated fat, plus they contain arginine, chromium, magnesium, phosphorous, selenium and Vitamin E. Most importantly for those who want to lose weight and gain a six-pack, nuts and seeds have vitamin B that enhances your metabolism and are rich in protein that helps build lean muscles.

Aside from that, nuts and seeds are a great source of fiber. This is important because foods that are high in fiber have less calorie content. Additionally, we tend to chew high fiber food longer, so we end up eating less as the brain has more time to process the fact that the stomach is already full. Foods that are high in fiber also take a longer time before it gets discharged from our system, thus, the feeling of fullness and satiation stays with your body longer.

Nuts and seeds are also known to contain generous portions of omega 3 fatty acids, a polyunsaturated fat that has anti-inflammatory properties, meaning you are protected against certain illnesses such as obesity.

They also support the body's capability to produce more energy, protect against aging and damage to cells, allow healthy formation of your skin, hair, nails, bones and teeth, ease blood flow by relaxing constricted blood vessels and guarding the walls of your arteries, and promote brain growth and development.

Nuts and seeds, however, are high in fat content and calorie level. So do take them in moderation. An ounce a day, which is around a handful, will do wonders for your health and your drive to lose weight.

Losing Weight by Going Green – The Magic of Green Tea

Green tea is a herbal product that can make the process of burning fat easier to achieve. That is because green tea contains an anti oxidant called polyphenols, which in turn has catechins, that can boost your metabolism and encourage your body to shed off your fat content. This herbal product also has caffeine that assists in the proper absorption of the catechins.

Green tea is especially effective for slightly obese and overweight individuals. While there is still a lot of research needed to definitely conclude the effectiveness of this product, there is absolutely no harm in trying it now. Consuming around 3 cups per day will help you in your quest to burn fat that will lead to ripped-up abs.

Red Hot Fat Burner – Spice Up with Chili Peppers

Chili peppers have an ingredient called capsaicin, which causes the body to heat up. Eating food spiced up with capsaicin allows the body to burn fat and calories for several more hours after its consumption. Food intake may decrease your calorie level by as much as 200 calories if it contains capsaicin. In addition, it may also cause a decrease in your appetite.

So do not hesitate to spice up your food like sandwiches, soups and eggs with capsaicin-powered chili peppers. It will not only add taste to your meals, it can also heat up you body and burn up the fat in your system.

9. Food You Must Avoid

Alcohol and Snacks

As a basic rule of thumb, one should keep away from sugar and salt if you want to lose weight and gain ripped abs. In particular, you must try to avoid alcohol and snacks.

Alcohol is merely refined juice. Its intake is like drinking concentrated sugar that will make you gain weight.

Snacks, on the other hand, can be addictive. So it will be wise to stay away from items like ice cream, cakes, popcorn, junk food, and the like. There are some healthy snack alternatives that you can try, and these were listed in Chapter 4.1.

Checking Out for Saturated Fat, Trans Fat and Sodium

There are basically three items in a food label that you must always have an eye out for – saturated fat, trans fat, and sodium level.

Saturated fat can increase your cholesterol level that will block your arteries and add to the risk of heart problems and cancer, so consumption must be kept at a low. Foods with significant saturated fat include red meat, butter, whole fat cheese, milk, dairy products, coconut oil and palm oil.

Trans fat can also increase the risk of heart disease. Avoid this totally by checking on the food label and making sure that the item carries zero trans fat. It is usually found in margarines, cakes, pies, and fried meals.

Sodium intake should be limited to a maximum of 2,400 mg per day. Too much sodium and the risk of heart attack increases. It can also lead to high blood pressure, and even a stroke and osteoporosis. Be wary of the sodium content of hot dogs, cheese, tomato sauce, canned soup, deli meat, frozen pizza, potato and pasta mixes and frozen microwave dinners.

Health Foods? – A Look at Unhealthy Health Food

Not all health foods are actually healthy. Some vegetables can basically contain only water with no nutrient value whatsoever. A primary example is iceberg lettuce. Enriched wheat flour may sound promising, but whole-wheat flour is the way to go as it is made up of 100% wheat. Adding the word multigrain does not necessarily mean a fibrous meal. Always check the food label for the amount of fiber included. And sea salt may sound so natural and health-friendly, but the bottom line is that its sodium content is practically the same as regular table salt.

10. Training and Exercise

While it is true that diet is the most important factor in losing weight and getting ripped abs, sustaining your ideal weight may be difficult to do if you do not engage yourself in regular workout training sessions that will help keep the fat away. Remember that to show off a six-pack, you have to make sure that there is no fat covering your belly.

Do not go crazy, however, by trying to train that belly fat off your abs. Spot training does not work, meaning it is not possible to lose fat in just one part of the body. To burn fat off, one must have a complete body workout.

5.1 Workouts

Pump Up Your Heart – Cardio Workouts

A cardio workout is the first training step towards achieving ripped up abs. Designed to increase your heart rate for a certain period of time, cardio workouts will help burn fat all over your body.

Cardio workouts can involve fun activities, such as running, swimming, cycling, rowing and even dancing. Even the simple jumping jacks or a brisk walk or jog are beneficial to your body. Aside from burning fat that will eventually lead to ripped-up abs, cardio workouts also actively train your arm and leg muscles.

You can also try to do some shadow boxing. Throw jabs, hooks and upper cuts, but control the manner of your punch. Do not flail or thrash around. Instead, focus by pretending that you have an opponent.

Ripping Up Without Too Much Equipment – Bodyweight Training Exercises

Some simple bodyweight workouts are actually the best way to attain a six-pack. Here are some bodyweight training exercises that you can easily do anytime and anywhere. You do not even have to go to the gym to do these exercises.

You can perform these exercises in a straight set format, meaning you should do 2 to 3 sets of each exercise, then resting for around 30 seconds in between each set. Alternatively, you can do the circuit format in which you will do all the exercises one after the other without any rest in between. Circuit must be done twice or thrice.

While it is true that diet is the most important factor in losing weight and getting ripped abs, sustaining your ideal weight may be difficult to do if you do not engage yourself in regular workout training sessions that will help keep the fat away. Remember that to show off a six-pack, you have to make sure that there is no fat covering your belly.

Do not go crazy, however, by trying to train that belly fat off your abs. Spot training does not work, meaning it is not possible to lose fat in just one part of the body. To burn fat off, one must have a complete body workout.

5.1 Workouts

Pump Up Your Heart – Cardio Workouts

A cardio workout is the first training step towards achieving ripped up abs. Designed to increase your heart rate for a certain period of time, cardio workouts will help burn fat all over your body.

Cardio workouts can involve fun activities, such as running, swimming, cycling, rowing and even dancing. Even the simple jumping jacks or a brisk walk or jog are beneficial to your body.

Aside from burning fat that will eventually lead to ripped-up abs, cardio workouts also actively train your arm and leg muscles.

You can also try to do some shadow boxing. Throw jabs, hooks and upper cuts, but control the manner of your punch. Do not flail or thrash around. Instead, focus by pretending that you have an opponent.

Ripping Up Without Too Much Equipment – Bodyweight Training Exercises

Some simple bodyweight workouts are actually the best way to attain a six-pack. Here are some bodyweight training exercises that you can easily do anytime and anywhere. You do not even have to go to the gym to do these exercises.

You can perform these exercises in a straight set format, meaning you should do 2 to 3 sets of each exercise, then resting for around 30 seconds in between each set. Alternatively, you can do the circuit format in which you will do all the exercises one after the other without any rest in between. Circuit must be done twice or thrice.

Workout sessions should be scheduled three to four times a week on non-consecutive days to allow your body to recover and your muscles to respond properly.

Bodyweight	How to Do It
Training Exercise	
Bicycle Crunches	Lie down while facing up.
	Put your hands behind your head, with the fingers lightly supporting your head.
	Raise your knees up to your chest.
	Lift your shoulders off the floor. Do not pull on the neck.

Rotate to the right so that your left elbow will touch your right knee, while you straighten up your left leg.
Rotate to the left side this time. Your right elbow should touch your left knee while your right leg straightens.
Keep pedaling by alternating sides.
Aim for 10 to 20 repetitions.
Sit down on a chair.
Keep your feet on the ground.
Lift your hips off the floor, putting all the weight on your hands.
Go back down slowly.
Aim for 10 to 20 repetitions.
On a flat and cushioned, but steady, surface, lie down flat on your back.
Knees should be at a 45-degree angle.
Fold your hands across the chest.
Sit up and roll your shoulders forward until they are 3 to 4 inches off the floor. The abs should do all the work.
Make sure that the small of your back remains in touch with the floor.
Count to 2.
Lie back slowly.
Aim for 10 to 20 repetitions.

Notes:

Crunches are not advisable to those suffering back pains.
Refrain from putting an anchor on your feet. It will just stress the back and the hips, and will also negate the abdominal gain that could have been achieved.
Do not lock your hands behind your neck to prevent stress.
This exercise will emphasize your upper abs.
Lie down on a slightly declined bench.
Hands should be holding the side of the bench.
Raise your pelvis and knees up to your chest.
Count to 2.
Lower the pelvis and knees back down.

Aim for 10 to 20 repetitions.

Chair Lift (requires a chair)
Crunches
Decline   Reverse Crunches

Notes:

Increase the decline of the bench if you want more resistance.
This exercise will emphasize your lower abs.
Lie down on the ball. Make sure that the ball is positioned right under your lower back.
Cross your arms over the chest.
Lift your torso off the ball. You should have the feeling of your lower ribs getting pulled down towards your hips.
Curl back up. The ball must be stable at all times.
Lower yourself down so that your abs will get stretched out.
Aim for 10 to 20 repetitions.
Lie down on a slightly declined bench.
Lock your feet on top of the bench.
Raise your hands so that it will slightly touch your head.
Pin your butt onto the bench.
Raise your body towards your knees while twisting your torso to the right side.
Count to 2.
Go back down.
Raise your body again towards your knees, but this time, twist your torso to the left side. Aim for 10 to 20 repetitions.

Note:

This exercise targets the oblique muscles.
Hang on to a chin up bar.
Raise your legs as high as you can, or if possible, until your knees touch your chest.
Hold for a count of 2.

Aim for 10 to 20 repetitions.

Lie on the mat with your face up.

Stretch out your arms behind your head such that the middle part of your arms will be right next to your ear.

Clasp your hands together.

Raise your shoulders off the floor while keeping the arms straight. Contract your abs while doing this.

Lower yourself back down slowly.

Aim for 10 to 20 repetitions.

Get into a push up position, either on your hands and toes or your elbows and toes.

Keep your back straight.

Contract the abdominal muscles.

Exercise Ball Crunch (requires an exercise ball)

Twisting Sit Ups

Leg   Raises

(requires a simple chin up bar where you can suspend yourself)

Long Arm Crunch

Plank Exercise

Hold it for as long as you can.

Aim for 3 to 5 repetitions.

Go into a sprinter's start position.

Straighten out your back.

Lift your right knee to your chest slowly.

Hold for a count of 2.

Lower your leg slowly, back to the start position.

Do the same with your left knee.

Do this for 45 seconds.

Lie straight on your right side with your right forearm propping up your upper body.

Make sure that the outer part of your right leg is the only part of your lower body touching the floor.

Raise your hips. Your body must form a straight line from your shoulders up to your ankles.

Contract the abdominal muscles.

Hold it for as long as you can.

Do the same with the left side of your body.

Aim for 3 to 5 repetitions.

Stand straight, feet slightly apart, and knees partly bent.

Hold a broom handle horizontally behind your neck.

Make sure that the center of the broom handle is resting at the base of your neck.

Twist your torso to the left.

Hold for a count of 2.

Now twist all the way around to the right.

Hold again for a 2 count.

Aim for 10 to 20 repetitions.

Lie down on the floor with the face up.

Extend your legs straight up so that it will form a 90-degree angle to your upper body.

Cross your knees.

You can place your hands behind your head, but do not pull on your neck.

Raise your shoulders off the floor. Try to reach your legs with your chest. Contract your abs while doing it.

Keep your legs steady. You should have a feeling of your belly button pushing down on your spine.

Get back down slowly.

Aim for 10 to 20 repetitions.

Mountain Climber

Side   Plank

Exercise

Standing Trunk Twist (requires a broom handle)

Vertical   Leg

Crunch

For those who do not have the time to do all the above listed exercises, here are samples of abs workout programs designed for different level of users.

Abs Workout for New Users

Do the following exercises one after the other, with 30 seconds of rest in between. Repeat two times.

- Plank exercise.
- Mountain Climber exercise.
- Side Plank exercise.

Abs Workout for Slightly Advanced Users

Slightly advanced users can do the same exercise routine as that of the new users, but with some slight variations. Again, do the following exercises one after the other, with 30 seconds of rest in between. Repeat two times.

- Plank exercise with feet on a bench.
- Mountain Climber exercise with hands on an exercise ball.
- Side Plank exercise with feet on a bench.

Abs Workout for the Advanced Hardcore Users

Option # 1

Do the following exercises one after the other, with 30 seconds of rest in between. Repeat two times.

- Plank exercise with the hands positioned around 7 to 8 inches in front of the shoulders.
- Mountain Climber exercise, with feet on an exercise ball trying to pull the ball forward.
- Side Plank exercise with the top leg raised into the air for the duration of the exercise.

Option # 2

You can also do this abs circuit by executing the following exercises one after the other without any rest in between. This will be done three times.

- Bicycle Crunch.
- Chair Lift.
- Exercise Ball Crunch.

Carry That Weight – Adding Further Resistance to Your Training Exercises

Abdominal exercises can be enhanced even more if you make use of weights or exercise balls. One of the keys in attaining six-pack abs is not by increasing the number of repetitions in your exercises, but by stiffening the resistance.

Carry a plate of weight when doing those crunches. Or strap in an ankle weight during the leg raise and mountain climbing exercise. Added resistance that will challenge your body even more will do wonders for your abs.

5.2 Training and Exercise Tips

How must one prepare for an exercise session? How intense should your training be? How often must it be conducted? Should this be done everyday?

Here are some helpful tips that you can use for your training session.

Warm Up Exercises

This is a must before the start of any training session. It prepares your muscles for more strenuous activities by increasing your heart and breathing rates, thus, minimizing the risk of an injury. It also increases the body's core temperature.

This should be done for 5 to 10 minutes, though a longer warm up session may be required for those residing in cold climates. Intensity should be gradually increased during the course of the warm up.

Training Intensity

The level of training intensity is based on your heart rate while doing the exercise. A person's maximum heart rate can be calculated by simply deducting your age from 220. Exercises that work up your heart rate to 65% of the maximum are defined as low intensity training. High intensity training, on the other hand, may work up your heart rate to as much as 85% of the maximum.

Low intensity training may actually burn more calories than high intensity exercises during the actual workout session. High intensity training, however, can boost your metabolism such that you will keep burning off calories even after you have finished with your exercises. Studies have also shown that high intensity training is more effective in burning off total abdominal fat, specifically subcutaneous abdominal fat, and abdominal visceral fat.

It is almost impossible to conduct and sustain a continuous session made up of purely high intensity exercises however. The most ideal thing to do is to have interval training workouts.

Interval training is very simple and very effective. It can be done with practically any cardio workout. Start off with a light warm-up cycle. You then move to a high intensity level for a short burst. You go back to a low level exercise for a while, and then back up again to a high level one. This is done several times before you taper off with a cooldown exercise. Each period may take as short as 30 seconds.

You can also utilize lower level exercises but with longer intervals. Bike around casually for a couple of minutes, and then pump those pedals furiously for 4 minutes. Or you can jog for 2 minutes, and alternate it with 3-minute runs. This is a good aerobic exercise as well.

Training Frequency

Determine first your overall goals before deciding on the frequency of your workout sessions. If you are aiming to build up your strength, then you will have to utilize stiffer resistance, like heavier weights or more inclined benches. That means that you will also need more time to recover, so training sessions can be scheduled around twice to thrice a week.

If you are after more stability for your core, you will have more exercises that will challenge your agility. Lesser weights will be required, so you will be able to exercise up to 4 times a week.

Lifting Tempo

In general, you need to let the weight down slower than when you raised it. The actual speed will depend on what you want to achieve.

If you want to increase the size of your muscles, concentrate on slow lifting. This will increase muscle tension that will help bulk up your mass.

On the other hand, focusing on a fast lifting speed will increase your power, thus allowing you to boost up your strength.

Repetitions

Train your abs muscle in the same way that you train the other muscles in your body. Do 2 to 3 sets of each exercise, with around

10 to 20 repetitions. If you do not feel tired after your training session, check out your form and see if you are doing things correctly.

You can also challenge yourself by doing new exercises. You can also train your abdominal muscles in a totally different way by trying out dynamic programs like Pilates.

Break Time in Between Sets

The break time in between your exercise sets is essential to your training program. Again, this will depend on what your goals are. If your goals require using stiffer resistance or heavier weights, then you can have fewer repetitions and longer time in between sets. Lifting lighter weights, on the other hand, require a shorter rest period even though it needs more repetitions.

Rest Days

For a training program to become effective, observing days of rest is essential to its success. Muscles require time to repair and recover.

11. Vitamin Supplements

Lose weight, gain life." "The miracle diet pill." "For every 2 pounds you lose, we will help you lose one more." "Pop the pill, burn the fat."

We have all read the promises and have gotten allured by their catch slogans. But do these fat loss supplements really help?

Below is a list of some of the more popular fat loss supplements available in the market. Again, always consult your physician before drinking any of these. And remember, the right nutrition plan and proper training exercises are still the ultimate fat burners.

Calcium Supplements

Calcium intake may be an effective tool in your drive to lose weight and shed off unwanted fat. Studies have shown that people who consume more calcium are less likely to become obese. It has been suggested that the brain will prompt hunger signals if it senses a deficiency of calcium in the system. Calcium also plays a role in resisting insulin and promoting a lean body mass.

The consumption (or non consumption) of this nutrient accounts for about a 3 to 10 percent difference in body weight. A thousand milligrams of calcium can mean as much as 18 pounds of difference.

The recommended daily allowance for calcium is 1,200 milligrams, which majority of the population do not get. Supplement as needed, preferably with a calcium nitrate taken once in the morning and another in the evening. This will let your body absorb the nutrient properly for maximum effectiveness and utilization and will allow you to avoid constipation and a feeling of being bloated. Avoid using coral calcium because it is known to contain impure ingredients.

Be careful not to go above 2,500 milligrams however. An overdose of calcium will make it difficult for your body to absorb zinc and iron, and this may lead to kidney stones. Too much calcium will also increase the risk of a heart attack.

Hydroxycut

Hydroxycut Hardcore is one of the most popular weight loss and fat burning supplement. The current Hydroxycut in the market is a reformulation of a previous product. The old Hydroxycut used to have the pride and distinction of being able to melt away your fat and dropping your weight by simply taking it in. Unfortunately, the reason for this is ephedrine, which has been banned as it has been proven to cause distress to the liver.

Hydroxycut has since removed ephedrine from its formulation. You will notice however that the new formulation comes with a caveat that it should be taken alongside a proper diet and training program for it to become effective. The only thing is, even without Hydroxycut, you can probably burn off a similar level of fat content and lose the same amount of weight if you just follow a disciplined nutrition and workout plan.

It is possible that Hydroxycut may give you some energy boost for your workout sessions as it contains elements of vitamin B. You should be wary of the caffeine content however as it may cause you anxiety and jitters.

Lipozene

Lipozene is an all-natural product that contains glucomannan, which is a water-soluble fiber extracted from the root of the konjac plant. It suppresses your appetite by giving you a feeling of satiation for a longer period of time.

Side effects that you might experience include diarrhea and a feeling of being bloated. There have also been reports of chest pain, vomiting, trouble in swallowing and difficulty in breathing. In extreme cases, there may be choking and blocking of the throat, esophagus and intestines unless you drink it with 8 ounces of water.

Lipozene may be effective, but adding foods that are rich in soluble fiber like oats, fruits, peas and beans to your meals will probably yield the same result.

Omega 3 Fatty Acids from Fish Oil

These are the good fat. Yes, you can fight fat with fat! Amazingly, those omega 3 fatty acids found in fish oil can actually burn your body's fat content. They have also been found to lower cholesterol and blood pressure and to reduce the risks of strokes and heart attacks.

Be sure to get from a reputable supplier, however, because there is always a danger of getting fish oil from fish that has not been tested for mercury. Also, excessive amounts of omega 3 fatty acids may increase the risk of bleeding.

Orlistat (Marketed as Xenical by Roche and as Alli by Glaxo Smith Kline)

The capsules that block fat. This is a drug that can make you lose weight by preventing the digestion and absorption of fat into your body. Orlistat does this by blocking the action of the enzyme that breaks down fat in your food. Your body does not absorb about 25% of the fat in your meal if you drink this capsule.

Orlistat should only be taken during or an hour after eating, and only if your meal has more than 15 mg of fat content.

There are downsides, of course. Your body may not absorb some nutrients properly if you take Orlistat, specifically those dietary vitamins that bind to fat. These are vitamin A, vitamin D, vitamin E and beta carotene. A multi vitamin containing these nutrients should be taken a couple of hours before or several hours after drinking the capsule.

An even worse downside is the mess that it could create. Its side effects include more bowel movements, an inability to control your stool, and even some oily spotting. It may also cause discomfort and pain to your abdomen.

There have also been cases of gall bladder and liver problems associated to the drinking of Orlistat.

Orlistat is the only weight loss and fat burning drug approved by the Food and Drug Administration. It is sold over the counter as Alli, and as a prescription drug with higher dosage as Xenical. Alli can help you lose additional weight of up to 3 to 5 pounds, while Xenical's higher dosage allows you to lose an additional weight of 5 to 7 pounds.

Phentermine

This drug works by suppressing your appetite and by stimulating your body so that you will increase the amount of energy you would use. It should not be taken alongside other appetite suppressants and must be used only as part of a short-term weight loss program.

That is because Phentermine may be addictive, so you should weigh the risks and benefits before popping it in. Once you have started, you may find it difficult to stop and be weaned away. Withdrawal symptoms might be experienced, meaning there will be bouts of depression and severe fatigue. Phentermine can also cause higher blood pressure, insomnia and even lung disorders if taken with other medications. Other side effects include blurred vision, constipation, dizziness, anxiety and dryness of the mouth.

Quick Trim Extreme Burn

The Kim Kardashian caplet. Bear in mind however that actresses with great curves probably have the benefit of good genes and good plastic surgeons.

This caplet contains a lot of ingredients, from caffeine to berries and cayenne pepper. If you take a balanced diet however, you can already get all the nutrients supplied by this caplet. The ingredients in Quick Trim Extreme Burn that do promote weight loss come in miniscule amounts that are not really enough for it to become effective.

Off Label Prescription Drugs

Some drugs that were originally intended for the treatment of other medical conditions can help a person lose weight. A physician must supervise when using these as part of a weight loss program however.

Examples of these are the following:

1. Wellbutrin – an anti depressant medication.
2. Metformin – an anti-diabetes drug.
3. Topiramate – an anti-seizure prescription.

6.3 Supplements That Help in Training and Muscle Building

These are the supplements that can help you build up your muscles by providing a boost during your workout sessions. There are a lot of supplements in the market that claim to have found a way to help in building bigger and stronger muscles, but these are the ones that really work.

Creatine

This one really works. The Creatine supplement will allow you to have explosive movements and will give you the power needed for a sudden burst of activity. Use this during high intensity training sessions, and you will find an increase in the strength of your muscles of up to 8% to 14%.

Creatine itself may help increase your muscle fibers. The added strength will also allow you to carry an additional weight load, which will lead to a bigger muscle size. Even better, taking Creatine will deplete the amount of lactic acid in your system, which means fatigue will become less of a factor during your training exercises as you will be able to recover within a shorter amount of time. Muscle pain also becomes more manageable after a strenuous workout session.

The only noticeable side effect of this supplement is the weight that you might gain. Take note however that the additional poundage is brought about by an increase in muscle mass, so it's not really a bad thing.

Creatine can also provide a boost to your mental capacity. It is also known to help those who are having sleep problems. And we have learned in chapter 3 that sleeping plays an essential role in the fat burning process.

For best results, take Creatine in powder form in servings of 10 grams twice a day for 2 days. Starting on the third day, continue the supplement with a maintenance dosage of 2 grams per day. Creatine is also available in pills, as well as in candy and gum forms in case these are more convenient for you to use. But do not take the liquid Creatine as it is not stable for long periods.

It is also advisable to consume carbohydrates when taking Creatine as insulin is needed for the supplement to be absorbed efficiently by the body. A better absorption rate means there will be more Creatine available for your muscles.

This supplement is not recommended however to those who have problems with their kidneys.

L-Glutamine

Glutamine is the most abundant amino acid found in our muscles and plasma. It plays a major role in our body's metabolism of protein and helps the body recover after an extremely tough workout session.

The natural glutamine in our body is consumed after a very physical training exercise. To compensate for this, the body sources glutamine from our muscles. As much as 40% of the muscle's glutamine gets depleted and as a result, muscle tissues will break down.

Taking L-Glutamine assures that our body has an available supply of this amino acid for our muscles, thus preventing the breakdown of muscle tissues. It also helps distribute nitrogen all over the body, which is needed in the building up of muscles.

L-Glutamine is also known to boost up a person's plasma human growth hormone (HGH) level. The increase in HGH will stimulate the anterior pituitary gland. The results are a lower level of fat in the body and a higher level of energy that will bring about a more intense training session. This will help in increasing your strength level and in further adding up to your muscle mass.

Other benefits of L-Glutamine include the enhancement of your digestive system as the cells in your intestinal tract will have higher absorption capacity, improvement in mental capacity, and augmentation of your immune system that will help counter infections in your body.

Take 10 grams of L-Glutamine right after your intense workout sessions to help your body recuperate quickly. You can also take 5 grams before you hit the sack to spike up your HGH level, and another serving right after waking up as your body has not taken in any nutrition during your sleeping hours.

If you are using anti-seizure medications, consult your doctor before taking this supplement.

Sports Drinks

Sports drinks are advisable for workouts in which the duration exceeds an hour, and even for shorter workouts that are intense and extremely physical. Water alone might not satisfy your needs and quench your thirst. For starters, water is tasteless. The flavor in a sports drink can help you keep on drinking, which is important as your body will need the fluid during those workout sessions.

12. Fakes, Hypes, Banned and Scams – Supplements That Must Be Avoided

Be careful when you buy your supplements. Not all of them work as well as advertised. They are just products of a creative and intelligent marketing campaign, with some of them making use of celebrities to feed the hype.

Some of them do not even work at all. They are the fake supplements that you can do without because its ingredients can be easily accessed by following a well-balanced and healthy nutrition plan.

The worst ones are the illegal supplements. These supplements have been banned, and for good reason. These substances have been found out to have really adverse side effects to the body. They are simply not worth it.

Below is a partial list of fake, hyped-up or illegal substances. You will do well in saving your money by avoiding these supplements.

Anabolic Steroids

Anabolic steroids duplicate the effects of testosterone and dihydrotestosterone. They increase protein synthesis and build up muscle tissues.

Anabolic steroids really work in helping a person bulk up, but this supplement produces plenty of side effects and is downright illegal. It is known to have harmful effects on the heart and liver and to have negative consequences to blood pressure and cholesterol levels. It has disgraced world famous athletes and got Ben Johnson kicked out of the Olympic Games.

Chitosan

Chitosan is a fiber supplement marketed as the ultimate fat trapper. It is a natural substance extracted from shellfish. Chitosan works by blocking the absorption of fats and getting rid of it from the digestive system. It is supposed to work just like Orlistat, specifically Xenical and Alli.

The downside is that it also blocks the proper absorption of other essential nutrients, specifically those vitamins that are soluble in fat (vitamin A, vitamin D, vitamin E, and vitamin K). It causes gastric problems to its users as well. Even worse, clinical studies have shown that the fat trapping claims of Chitosan are largely unsubstantiated.

Human Growth Hormone (HGH) Supplements

Human growth hormone (HGH) supplements can alter your body's composition by reducing your fat content and increasing your muscle mass. HGH supplements can also assist your performance in workout sessions because it can boost your energy level. Aside from increasing your muscle tone, HGH supplements can also supposedly improve your skin and the density of your bones.

You should be wary before trying out this supplement however. There have only been very few studies made to analyze the effects and dangers of HGH supplements. As it is, regular users are more likely to develop diabetes. It is also known to cause carpal tunnel syndrome, swelling of the joints and soft tissue edema. In the end, HGH supplements probably will not be able to deliver as much as they have touted to.

L-Carnitine

The L-Carnitine supplement has been marketed to improve endurance and to shorten the recovery time needed after a workout by rejuvenating your muscles. It takes the fatty acids you consumed with your meals and convert them to energy. L-Carnitine is said to have the ability to increase your vigor to a level so high that it would lead to an extremely intense training session.

L-Carnitine also serves as an anti-oxidant and can help mend your injuries. It also helps balance the function of your thyroid gland, thus enhancing your body's metabolism.

Numerous studies have been conducted, however, in various countries and most have yielded negative results. While L-Carnitine may have some benefits for fat oxidation, none of the studies have shown the supplement as having any impact that will increase your workout session performance, enhance your metabolism or alter your fat content and muscle mass.

Meridia

Meridia was a very common diet pill prescribed by doctors. It works by altering your brain function so that your appetite and cravings will be managed and controlled. Eventually, this will lead to less meal intake as you will have a feeling of fullness even if you have not consumed that much food.

There were findings however of Meridia causing breakdowns in its users' heart and liver. It was subsequently taken off the market in the latter part of 2010.

Prohormones

A prohormone is a precursor to an actual hormone. It is a supplement that works by giving out a signal to your body to release more hormones that you can use to gain strength, to enable fast muscle recovery and to promote muscle growth.

Prohormones came about as a result of the banning of anabolic steroids. Its effects were the same as anabolic steroids as users experienced increase in strength, power, muscle mass and recovery.

Using it may cause adverse side effects. Prohormones have been found to cause extreme damage to the prostrate and liver. It can also affect your blood pressure.

In 2004, a significant percentage of prohormones were found to have ingredients similar to anabolic steroids. They were subsequently included in the list of banned substances.

Pyruvate

Pyruvate is produced when the body breaks down sugar. It is also available as a supplement and is reputed to help a person who wants to lose weight by breaking down the body's fat content. It is also said to provide a boost for training exercise sessions as it increases a user's endurance level.

Studies have shown however that for Pyruvate to work properly, you will need to consume around 50 capsules per day. This borders on a scam, as it will put a major dent not only on your stomach but also on your savings.

13. Conclusion

So the beach outing is just a week away, and you have yet to attain that six-pack. No more use crying over spilled milk and thinking of what you could have achieved had you started your quest for a six-pack months ago.

But you can always try to go on a crash course or an expedited fast track abs training program. While there is no guarantee that you will get the desired washboard of those models in fitness magazines, there is also no harm in trying.

The presumption here, of course, is that you are at least physically fit and only a few pounds above your recommended weight level. If you are way above the recommended weight range, ripping up your abs in just 7 days may be an impossible task.

 If you are indeed physically fit who can stand the rigors of an extremely intensive and physical training week and who possess the commitment and the discipline to follow through on a challenging nutrition plan, then you may try to do the steps outlined below that can lead to ripped up abs within one week.

A note of caution is needed however. You should not attempt the following nutrition and training exercise plan for an amount of time longer than seven days.

1.	This is an extreme diet plan that should only be followed for this special crash course abs training program. The plan is to basically cut all the carbohydrates from your meals and to consume the smallest amount of fat possible. Your meal intakes will be practically made up of pure protein. That means unseasoned and tasteless white meat from poultry products like chicken or turkey.

What it will do is the body will have no other choice but to use up its storage of fat and convert it to energy. There might be some fatigue that will be experienced while doing this, mainly because of the absence of other nutrients in the body, and also because of the bland protein meal you are consuming. You need to get past this obstacle however, as you will need to channel a lot of energy for the workout sessions.

2.   Keep doing cardio workouts. Bike and run and swim beyond the point of exhaustion. The idea here is to create a calorie deficit by burning more than you have taken in. Combining this with the extreme diet that you are following, and you will lose weight faster than ever.

3.   Pump up those irons. Add more resistance to your abs workout. When doing crunches, carry a plate of weight across your chest for more challenge. Once you get used to it, add some more poundage. You can also strap on some ankle weights when doing leg raise and mountain climber exercises. You can also try steeper angles when doing sit-ups and crunches.

4.   Make sure that you have the right supplements. As discussed in chapter six, supplements can help you get over the top. Load up on Creatine for more bursts of power and L-Glutamine for faster recovery and for proper buildup of your muscles. Whey protein should also be consumed. Whey protein concentrates, however, have a lesser amount of protein and contain some carbohydrates and calories. Get whey protein isolate instead. Isolate is better than concentrate because it has 90% pure protein and practically no carbohydrates and minimal calories.

5.   Remain active at all times possible. Remember that you want to burn off as much fat and calories as you can. So be on the move all the time. Do some brisk walking or climb some stairs in between your workout training schedules. Or do some laps on the swimming pool or bike around the neighborhood.

6.	Consume a lot of water. This will ensure that your body remains hydrated all the time. It will also give you a feeling of fullness while not adding up to your calorie level.

7.	As discussed in chapter three, sleep is an important and essential factor in losing weight, burning fat, and getting six-pack abs. Make sure that you get enough shut eye time during this one week training program. Seven to eight hours of sleep will provide your body with enough rest for your muscles to recover.

Through all this, keep an eye on your ultimate goal of achieving rock hard washboard abs in a week. That thought alone may be enough to strengthen your commitment to this extreme one-week nutrition and training program. It will not be easy and there will be a number of times when you will think of quitting, but a possible six-pack is waiting for you if you complete this weeklong abs-building program.

www.ingramcontent.com/pod-product-compliance
Lightning Source LLC
Chambersburg PA
CBHW030534290526
45786CB00004B/1715